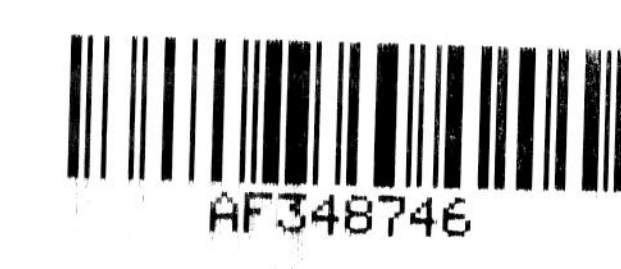

Made in the USA
Monee, IL
07 July 2026

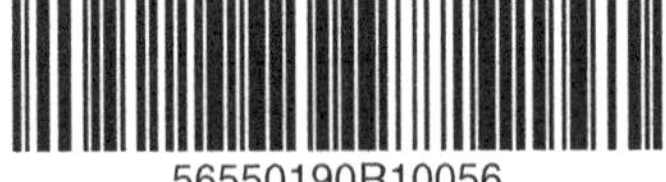